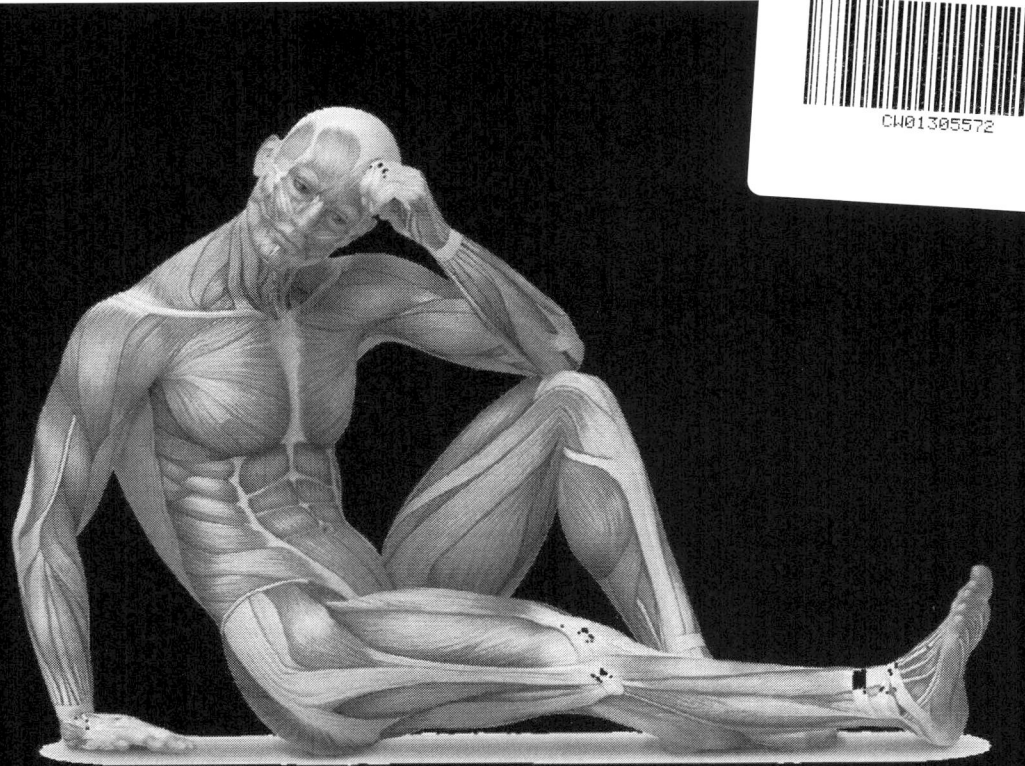

ANATOMY CHEAT SHEETS

The Easiest Way to Learn Human Parts

70 Terms & Def	Quiz	Matching
Test	Word Search	Crosswords
BINGO	Table Review	Quick Study

Anatomy Table Review

Anatomy

Definition	Term
tarsal	ankle
orbital	eye
femoral	thigh
thoracic cavity location	encircled by ribs, sternum, vertebral column, muscle divided into two pleural cavities by mediastinum
facial	face
keratinocyte distinguish	intermediate filament, keratin
merkel cell distinguish	tactile, Merkel disc
tissue level integument	stratum corneum, dead keratinocytes, stratum lucidum, stratum granulosum, lamellar granules, stratum spinosum, langerhans cell, melanocytes, stratum basale, merkel cell, tactile disc, sensory neuron, dermis, blood vessel
antecubital	front of elbow
loin	lumbar
olecranal	back of elbow
Tissues	epithelial, connective, muscle, nervous
umbilical	navel
trunk	abdomen are
popliteal	hollow behind knee
dorsal	back
Anatomical	standing upright, facing the observer, eyes facing forward, feet flat on floor, arms at sides, palms turned forward
pedal	foot
Cellular level integument	keratinocyte, melanocyte, langerhans cell, merkel cell, sensory neuron
thoracic cavity organs right side, anterior to posterior	sternum, muscle, pericardium, right lung, right pleura, esophagus, sixth thoracic vertebra, right pleural cavity, rib
scapular	shoulder lade
cervical	neck
crural	leg
Supine	lying face up
Epithelial	covers surfaces because cells are in contact, lines hollow organs, cavities and ducts, forms glands when cells sink under the surface
dorsum	back of hand
acromial	shoulder
inguinal	groin
coxal	hip
cephalic	head
sural	calf
Systemic Anatomy	organization of body into organ systems

	definition
sternal	breastbone
thoracic	chest
occipital	base of skull
cranial	skull
digital	fingers
nasal	nose
dorsum	top of foot
mental	chin
posterior	towards the back
sacral	between hips
anterior	towards the front
melanocyte distinguish	melanin granule
thoracic cavity organs left side, anterior to posterior	thymus gland, heart, pericardial cavity, left lung, horaic aorta, left pleural cavity, scapula
manual	hand
mediastinum's organs	thymus gland, heart, pericardial cavity, thoracic aorta, left pleural cavity, scapula, sternum, muscle, pericardium, right pleura, esophagus, sixth thoracic veertebra, rib
oral	mouth
plantar	sole
brachial	arm
calcaneal	heel
abdominopelvic cavity organs	liver, diaphragm, stomach, gallbladder, large intestine, abdominal cavity, pelvic cavity, small intestine, urinary bladder
patellar	anterior surface of knee
digital	toes
integumentary system	dermal papilla, capillary loop, sweat pore, sebaceous gland, meissner copuscle, arrector pili muscle, hair follicle, hair root, eccrine sweat gland, pacinian corpuscle, sensory nerve, adipose tissue, vein, artery
Systemic Anatomy	integumentary, skeletal, muscular, articular, nervous, circulatory, digestive, respiratory, urinary, reproductive, endocrine
phalangeal	fingers or toes
axillary	armpit
buccal	cheek
otic	ear
antebrachial	forearm
vertebral	spinal column
Connective	tissues that bind together; cells rarely touch due to extracellular matrix; matrix (fibers & ground substance secreted by cells), consistency varies: liquid, gel, &solid; Doesn't occur on free surface, good nerve & blood supply except cartilage & tendons
carpal	wrist
abdominopelvic cavity location	inferior portion of ventral body cavity below diaphragm encircled by abdominal wall, bones, and muscles of pelvis
frontal	head
Prone	lying face down
palmar	palm

Anatomy Definition Flashcards

Terms on EVEN Pages and Definition on ODD Pages

Systemic Anatomy definition	Epithelial
Systemic Anatomy	Connective
Tissues	Anatomical
Supine	Prone

covers surfaces because cells are in contact, lines hollow organs, cavities and ducts,	organization of body into organ systems
tissues that bind together; cells rarely touch due to extracellular matrix; matrix (fibers &	integumentary, skeletal, muscular, articular, nervous, circulatory, digestive,
standing upright, facing the observer, eyes facing forward, feet flat on floor, arms at sides, palms	epithelial, connective, muscle, nervous
lying face down	lying face up

cephalic	facial
cranial	frontal
occipital	orbital
buccal	otic

face	head
head	skull
eye	base of skull
ear	cheek

nasal	cervical
oral	thoracic
mental	sternal
coxal	umbilical

neck	nose
chest	mouth
breastbone	chin
navel	hip

inguinal	acromial
trunk	scapular
dorsal	vertebral
brachial	axillary

shoulder	groin
shoulder lade	abdomen are
spinal column	back
armpit	arm

antecubital	carpal
olecranal	manual
antebrachial	dorsum
digital	palmar

wrist	front of elbow
hand	back of elbow
back of hand	forearm
palm	fingers

phalangeal	femoral
loin	patellar
sacral	popliteal
sural	crural

thigh	fingers or toes
anterior surface of knee	lumbar
hollow behind knee	between hips
leg	calf

pedal	dorsum
tarsal	plantar
digital	calcaneal
abdominopelvic cavity organs	abdominopelvic cavity location

top of foot	foot
sole	ankle
heel	toes
inferior portion of ventral body cavity below diaphragm encircled by abdominal wall,	liver, diaphragm, stomach, gallbladder, large intestine, abdominal cavity, pelvic

thoracic cavity location	anterior
mediastinum's organs	posterior
thoracic cavity organs left side, anterior to posterior	thoracic cavity organs right side, anterior to posterior
tissue level integument	integumentary system

towards the front	encircled by ribs, sternum, vertebral column, muscle divided into two pleural cavities by
towards the back	thymus gland, heart, pericardial cavity, thoracic aorta, left pleural cavity, scapula, sternum,
sternum, muscle, pericardium, right lung, right pleura, esophagus, sixth thoracic vertebra,	thymus gland, heart, pericardial cavity, left lung, horaic aorta, left pleural cavity, scapula
dermal papilla, capillary loop, sweat pore, sebaceous gland, meissner copuscle,	stratum corneum, dead keratinocytes, stratum lucidum, stratum granulosum,

Cellular level integument	merkel cell distinguish
keratinocyte distinguish	
melanocyte distinguish	

tactile, Merkel disc	keratinocyte, melanocyte, langerhans cell, merkel cell, sensory neuron
	intermediate filament, keratin
	melanin granule

Anatomy Definitions Flashcards Activities

Anatomy Word Search Puzzle

```
K V L A I H C A R B E T N A L A T I P I C C O O P D A E L S V V X G F
T S E J Q P L S L P O S T E R I O R B I T A L L O R X U U L A R U S A
J A B R O R T A S A B J K S E U S S I T N R X A A C A P U L L M C B P
R B R C T E A F N V C U U M B I L I C A L G E E Q T I P A E N E E P O
I Z B S R E E T C A P I C Y C F R O N T A L U T C N I I Q V I U P H R
S M Z N A A B Q N I R S M C L A S R O D W Y M I E C B T I O S H A S U
J W A O K L L R I A C C L O A Y R F E M O R A L N A T U U T L P A L M
M L A I N A R C A P L A E C T L I P Y S P I A P F A N O L C J M L A N
B R A C H I A L G L E P R L R A L U A T G T B O H Y L Z A E E E I N C
W R O I R E T N A N W U L O O U N Z V L X A Z P K H N G S N F T C G S
S X C E R V I C A L B L L K H E R A V J P A L M A R O C A N H V N E O
D I G I T A L C K P B A P E N T E A L A U N A M B I Y R N O I D A A I
E P I T H E L I A L F R N L A D E P L X N C A V I T Y L A C U G N L O
H Y M O T A N A C I M E T S Y S P A T E L L A R I Q C O A L X J Q F D
H E B C C J S Z A C R O M I A L N Y C O X A L X S V F U A F L L U J H
```

- ☐ FEMORAL
- ☐ POPLITEAL
- ☐ DIGITAL
- ☐ PALMAR
- ☐ SURAL
- ☐ SCAPULAR
- ☐ PLANTAR
- ☐ SUPINE
- ☐ EPITHELIAL
- ☐ ANTEBRACHIAL
- ☐ CARPAL
- ☐ PHALANGEAL
- ☐ SACRAL
- ☐ PEDAL
- ☐ BUCCAL
- ☐ NASAL
- ☐ ORBITAL
- ☐ ANTECUBITAL
- ☐ CONNECTIVE
- ☐ INGUINAL
- ☐ VERTEBRAL
- ☐ STERNAL
- ☐ ANATOMICAL
- ☐ TARSAL
- ☐ ANTERIOR
- ☐ CRANIAL
- ☐ FACIAL
- ☐ POSTERIOR
- ☐ OTIC
- ☐ CALCANEAL
- ☐ CEPHALIC
- ☐ FRONTAL
- ☐ LOIN
- ☐ CRURAL
- ☐ CERVICAL
- ☐ COXAL
- ☐ SYSTEMIC ANATOMY
- ☐ ORAL
- ☐ CAVITY
- ☐ DORSUM
- ☐ BRACHIAL
- ☐ ACROMIAL
- ☐ UMBILICAL
- ☐ MANUAL
- ☐ TISSUES
- ☐ OLECRANAL
- ☐ THORACIC
- ☐ OCCIPITAL
- ☐ DORSAL
- ☐ PATELLAR

Anatomy Word Search Puzzle

```
T Z P W E G F R T L A M E L L A R L U M B A R F S T O M A C H G L L A
P R X E R O I E C A F R U S U Y N T Z K W L R B O T H I G H T K K Y E
A H I O V T N P O N M O U T H E I Q I U H O S R F O N T F V O S C I L
N M I D D R G V T I A U X S C M A N F P K T B T E R T E O Y P U A N U
B N D C C E E Z L H T O R K J P J T G A M P A L M C Y P R Q O R B G N
H E A D U S R J K C H E S T S O K X M F G R I F E V T A W N F F E F A
C F B Y P O S A Q Z G L L U K S F O E S A B A J O F N O A V F A H A R
A K I A I N O N N N B R E A S T B O N E V C J Q M I O J R N O C T C G
V F E L C N R V I E L H J E K L M J F C V Q E Y R K Y T D R O E S E N
I R C E A K T F L R M S T S C R M V L N F Y E U E W I A N S T M D D I
T B F V H M O E Y M F O K X A A D X A A N K L E P I G X I O P T R O N
Y S W Z I C E E O F N U D E U G F B C N W X H N A V E L Z B R Q A W A
V Q B Q L H S N E W L M R B H O L L O W B E H I N D K N E E U F W N L
C A H I T Y E X T L M O H M A T N O R F E H T S D R A W O T Y U O D E
P H E A D Z S O L E F Q S W R I S T N M B A C K O F H A N D W R T Y M
```

- BACK
- FRONT OF ELBOW
- BACK OF HAND
- ABDOMEN ARE
- FOOT
- CHIN
- FINGERS
- PALM
- FILAMENT
- LAMELLAR
- THIGH
- CAVITY
- TOP OF FOOT
- SURFACE
- ARMPIT
- CAVITY
- LYING FACE UP
- BREASTBONE
- HEEL
- CALF
- FOREARM
- SOLE
- CHEEK
- HEAD
- TOWARDS THE FRONT
- URINARY
- LYING FACE DOWN
- MELANIN GRANULE
- HEAD
- ANKLE
- WRIST
- NECK
- FINGERS OR TOES
- FACE
- NAVEL
- ARRECTOR
- NOSE
- SKULL
- HOLLOW BEHIND KNEE
- BASE OF SKULL
- TOWARDS THE BACK
- STOMACH
- GROIN
- SURFACE
- CHEST
- MOUTH
- LUMBAR
- FORWARD

B I N G O

cranial	manual	otic	dorsum	antecubital
palmar	integumentary system	thoracic cavity organs left side, anterior to posterior	sacral	nasal
crural	calcaneal	FREE	merkel cell distinguish	trunk
Systemic Anatomy definition	thoracic	occipital	pedal	patellar
plantar	tarsal	digital	femoral	posterior

B I N G O

B	I	N	G	O
keratinocyte distinguish	coxal	digital	trunk	facial
sacral	frontal	antebrachial	nasal	otic
cervical	melanocyte distinguish	FREE	thoracic cavity organs right side, anterior to posterior	abdominopelvic cavity organs
Cellular level integument	mental	carpal	umbilical	phalangeal
Epithelial	axillary	manual	pedal	palmar

BINGO

B	I	N	G	O
thoracic cavity location	calcaneal	Systemic Anatomy definition	integumentary system	Supine
anterior	pedal	vertebral	carpal	dorsum
Systemic Anatomy	loin	FREE	mediastinum's organs	melanocyte distinguish
dorsum	acromial	digital	tarsal	cephalic
manual	abdominopelvic cavity organs	Prone	dorsal	Epithelial

BINGO

B	I	N	G	O
dorsum	merkel cell distinguish	antecubital	vertebral	inguinal
facial	calcaneal	keratinocyte distinguish	Systemic Anatomy definition	thoracic cavity organs right side, anterior to posterior
tissue level integument	mental	FREE	dorsum	patellar
digital	Supine	digital	thoracic cavity organs left side, anterior to posterior	crural
anterior	pedal	Systemic Anatomy	posterior	thoracic

B	I	N	G	O
popliteal	phalangeal	olecranal	axillary	Cellular level integument
thoracic cavity organs right side, anterior to posterior	buccal	dorsum	nasal	crural
facial	integumentary system	FREE	cephalic	Prone
patellar	tarsal	Systemic Anatomy	posterior	sural
coxal	manual	thoracic	otic	plantar

B	I	N	G	O
nasal	brachial	thoracic cavity organs right side, anterior to posterior	calcaneal	thoracic cavity organs left side, anterior to posterior
otic	sural	manual	buccal	digital
Prone	coxal	FREE	sacral	umbilical
antebrachial	cranial	Connective	dorsum	Supine
plantar	posterior	occipital	patellar	sternal

B	I	N	G	O
plantar	inguinal	mediastinum's organs	thoracic	mental
posterior	carpal	trunk	manual	Epithelial
axillary	integumentary system	FREE	melanocyte distinguish	Systemic Anatomy definition
antecubital	oral	coxal	cranial	thoracic cavity organs right side, anterior to posterior
calcaneal	Systemic Anatomy	nasal	acromial	phalangeal

B	I	N	G	O
brachial	crural	antebrachial	sural	posterior
calcaneal	cervical	nasal	orbital	integumentary system
thoracic	occipital	FREE	facial	vertebral
Supine	otic	keratinocyte distinguish	sacral	acromial
Connective	loin	femoral	anterior	inguinal

B	I	N	G	O
Supine	thoracic cavity organs left side, anterior to posterior	calcaneal	dorsal	sural
Anatomical	inguinal	Systemic Anatomy definition	patellar	mental
abdominopelvic cavity location	umbilical	FREE	cervical	scapular
pedal	popliteal	orbital	cranial	frontal
trunk	plantar	oral	merkel cell distinguish	Connective

B	I	N	G	O
digital	integumentary system	tarsal	melanocyte distinguish	coxal
calcaneal	Supine	crural	scapular	thoracic
cranial	mental	FREE	mediastinum's organs	Cellular level integument
posterior	olecranal	manual	frontal	axillary
patellar	occipital	trunk	otic	loin

B	I	N	G	O
thoracic	calcaneal	abdominopelvic cavity organs	Systemic Anatomy definition	dorsal
olecranal	keratinocyte distinguish	occipital	cranial	abdominopelvic cavity location
mediastinum's organs	otic	FREE	phalangeal	popliteal
integumentary system	crural	tarsal	umbilical	mental
femoral	antebrachial	antecubital	merkel cell distinguish	inguinal

B I N G O

manual	melanocyte distinguish	inguinal	tarsal	cranial
posterior	merkel cell distinguish	orbital	pedal	anterior
integumentary system	umbilical	FREE	trunk	facial
thoracic cavity location	Connective	dorsum	femoral	axillary
patellar	thoracic	Epithelial	popliteal	mental

B I N G O

B	I	N	G	O
digital	Epithelial	otic	thoracic cavity organs left side, anterior to posterior	sternal
manual	orbital	abdominopelvic cavity organs	coxal	calcaneal
antecubital	tissue level integument	FREE	pedal	frontal
mediastinum's organs	digital	Systemic Anatomy	patellar	vertebral
Anatomical	inguinal	olecranal	cranial	keratinocyte distinguish

B I N G O

vertebral	integumentary system	dorsum	acromial	sternal
Systemic Anatomy definition	keratinocyte distinguish	popliteal	dorsum	otic
cervical	abdominopelvic cavity location	FREE	thoracic cavity organs left side, anterior to posterior	buccal
occipital	cranial	sural	Tissues	antecubital
Anatomical	facial	tarsal	thoracic cavity location	palmar

B	I	N	G	O
Systemic Anatomy	scapular	trunk	plantar	calcaneal
tarsal	cervical	cephalic	tissue level integument	Cellular level integument
abdominopelvic cavity location	brachial	FREE	abdominopelvic cavity organs	digital
frontal	inguinal	patellar	thoracic	Connective
integumentary system	posterior	crural	oral	Anatomical

B	I	N	G	O
nasal	occipital	abdominopelvic cavity location	cephalic	brachial
sternal	plantar	crural	integumentary system	inguinal
keratinocyte distinguish	digital	FREE	tarsal	mental
coxal	melanocyte distinguish	axillary	otic	Connective
popliteal	loin	sacral	mediastinum's organs	cervical

B	I	N	G	O
otic	anterior	popliteal	mediastinum's organs	sacral
oral	Connective	buccal	dorsal	Anatomical
trunk	Systemic Anatomy definition	FREE	thoracic cavity location	olecranal
keratinocyte distinguish	mental	palmar	posterior	orbital
plantar	sternal	Epithelial	calcaneal	femoral

BINGO

B	I	N	G	O
mediastinum's organs	coxal	popliteal	facial	mental
digital	vertebral	manual	Cellular level integument	olecranal
palmar	Systemic Anatomy	FREE	tarsal	patellar
Epithelial	buccal	inguinal	Supine	cephalic
thoracic cavity location	merkel cell distinguish	sacral	integumentary system	abdominopelvic cavity location

B I N G O

B	I	N	G	O
Supine	Systemic Anatomy	trunk	patellar	integumentary system
acromial	cephalic	Cellular level integument	olecranal	phalangeal
dorsal	cervical	FREE	abdominopelvic cavity organs	oral
melanocyte distinguish	femoral	axillary	keratinocyte distinguish	anterior
mediastinum's organs	occipital	scapular	thoracic cavity location	thoracic

	B	I	N	G	O
	facial	popliteal	inguinal	tarsal	thoracic cavity location
	dorsal	dorsum	phalangeal	cephalic	Connective
	plantar	dorsum	FREE	cervical	loin
	carpal	mental	Prone	palmar	otic
	thoracic	buccal	Supine	umbilical	femoral

B	I	N	G	O	
B	I	N	G	O	organization of body into organ systems
B	I	N	G	O	integumentary, skeletal, muscular, articular, nervous, circulatory, digestive, respiratory, urinary, reproductive, endocrine
B	I	N	G	O	epithelial, connective, muscle, nervous
B	I	N	G	O	covers surfaces because cells are in contact, lines hollow organs, cavities and ducts, forms glands when cells sink under the surface
B	I	N	G	O	tissues that bind together; cells rarely touch due to extracellular matrix; matrix (fibers & ground substance secreted by cells), consistency varies: liquid, gel, &solid; Doesn't occur on free surface, good nerve & blood supply except cartilage & tendons
B	I	N	G	O	standing upright, facing the observer, eyes facing forward, feet flat on floor, arms at sides, palms turned forward
B	I	N	G	O	lying face down
B	I	N	G	O	lying face up
B	I	N	G	O	head
B	I	N	G	O	skull
B	I	N	G	O	base of skull
B	I	N	G	O	face
B	I	N	G	O	head
B	I	N	G	O	eye
B	I	N	G	O	ear
B	I	N	G	O	cheek
B	I	N	G	O	nose
B	I	N	G	O	mouth
B	I	N	G	O	chin
B	I	N	G	O	neck
B	I	N	G	O	chest
B	I	N	G	O	breastbone
B	I	N	G	O	navel
B	I	N	G	O	hip
B	I	N	G	O	groin
B	I	N	G	O	abdomen are
B	I	N	G	O	back
B	I	N	G	O	shoulder
B	I	N	G	O	shoulder lade
B	I	N	G	O	spinal column
B	I	N	G	O	armpit
B	I	N	G	O	arm
B	I	N	G	O	front of elbow
B	I	N	G	O	back of elbow
B	I	N	G	O	forearm
B	I	N	G	O	wrist
B	I	N	G	O	hand
B	I	N	G	O	back of hand
B	I	N	G	O	palm
B	I	N	G	O	fingers
B	I	N	G	O	fingers or toes
B	I	N	G	O	lumbar

B	I	N	G	O	
B	I	N	G	O	between hips
B	I	N	G	O	thigh
B	I	N	G	O	anterior surface of knee
B	I	N	G	O	hollow behind knee
B	I	N	G	O	leg
B	I	N	G	O	calf
B	I	N	G	O	foot
B	I	N	G	O	ankle
B	I	N	G	O	toes
B	I	N	G	O	top of foot
B	I	N	G	O	sole
B	I	N	G	O	heel
B	I	N	G	O	inferior portion of ventral body cavity below diaphragm encircled by abdominal wall, bones, and muscles of pelvis
B	I	N	G	O	liver, diaphragm, stomach, gallbladder, large intestine, abdominal cavity, pelvic cavity, small intestine, urinary bladder
B	I	N	G	O	encircled by ribs, sternum, vertebral column, muscle divided into two pleural cavities by mediastinum
B	I	N	G	O	thymus gland, heart, pericardial cavity, thoracic aorta, left pleural cavity, scapula, sternum, muscle, pericardium, right pleura, esophagus, sixth thoracic veertebra, rib
B	I	N	G	O	thymus gland, heart, pericardial cavity, left lung, horaic aorta, left pleural cavity, scapula
B	I	N	G	O	towards the front
B	I	N	G	O	towards the back
B	I	N	G	O	sternum, muscle, pericardium, right lung, right pleura, esophagus, sixth thoracic vertebra, right pleural cavity, rib
B	I	N	G	O	dermal papilla, capillary loop, sweat pore, sebaceous gland, meissner copuscle, arrector pili muscle, hair follicle, hair root, eccrine sweat gland, pacinian corpuscle, sensory nerve, adipose tissue, vein, artery
B	I	N	G	O	stratum corneum, dead keratinocytes, stratum lucidum, stratum granulosum, lamellar granules, stratum spinosum, langerhans cell, melanocytes, stratum basale, merkel cell, tactile disc, sensory neuron, dermis, blood vessel
B	I	N	G	O	keratinocyte, melanocyte, langerhans cell, merkel cell, sensory neuron
B	I	N	G	O	intermediate filament, keratin
B	I	N	G	O	melanin granule
B	I	N	G	O	tactile, Merkel disc

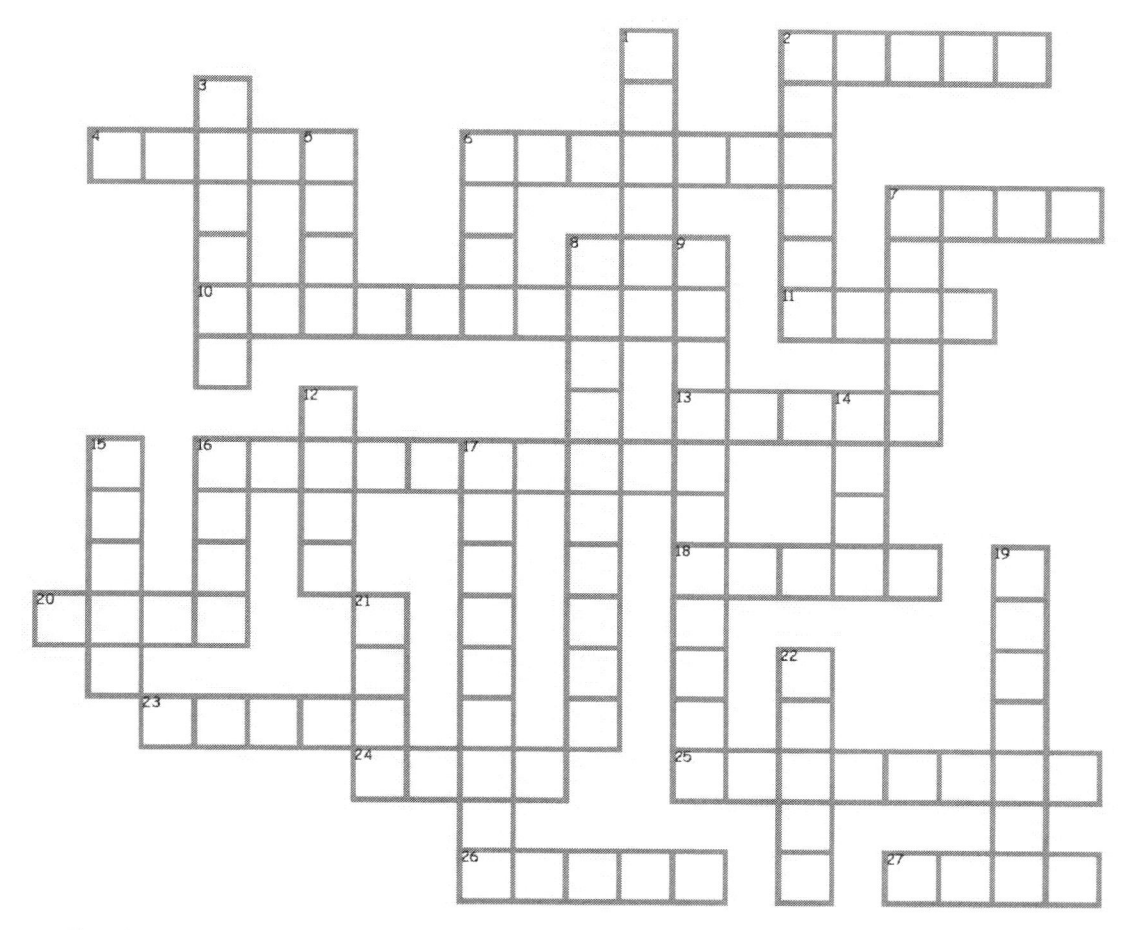

Across
- 2 tarsal
- 4 oral
- 6 antebrachial
- 7 mental
- 10 trunk
- 11 digital
- 13 carpal
- 16 sternal
- 18 umbilical
- 20 cervical
- 23 cranial
- 24 pedal
- 25 acromial
- 26 femoral
- 27 nasal

Down
- 1 calcaneal
- 2 axillary
- 3 loin
- 5 manual
- 6 facial
- 7 thoracic
- 8 dorsum
- 9 sacral
- 12 cephalic
- 14 plantar
- 15 buccal
- 16 dorsal
- 17 dorsum
- 19 digital
- 21 sural
- 22 inguinal

Anatomy Matching

Write the code corresponding to the correct match in the space provided.

___ 1. antebrachial
___ 2. sural
___ 3. vertebral
___ 4. Prone
___ 5. popliteal
___ 6. sacral
___ 7. tarsal
___ 8. thoracic cavity location
___ 9. nasal
___ 10. dorsum
___ 11. integumentary system
___ 12. loin
___ 13. brachial
___ 14. sternal
___ 15. axillary
___ 16. patellar
___ 17. thoracic cavity organs right side, anterior to posterior
___ 18. thoracic
___ 19. frontal
___ 20. Tissues
___ 21. cranial
___ 22. Supine
___ 23. umbilical
___ 24. coxal
___ 25. digital
___ 26. carpal
___ 27. cephalic
___ 28. antecubital
___ 29. Epithelial
___ 30. oral
___ 31. keratinocyte distinguish

A1. tactile, Merkel disc
B1. foot
C1. abdomen are
D1. head
E1. organization of body into organ systems
F1. stratum corneum, dead keratinocytes, stratum lucidum, stratum granulosum, lamellar granules, stratum spinosum, langerhans cell, melanocytes, stratum basale, merkel cell, tactile disc, sensory neuron, dermis, blood vessel
G1. epithelial, connective, muscle, nervous
H1. ear
I1. arm
J1. head
K1. lying face up
L1. hip
M1. top of foot
N1. toes
O1. lying face down
P1. dermal papilla, capillary loop, sweat pore, sebaceous gland, meissner copuscle, arrector pili muscle, hair follicle, hair root, eccrine sweat gland, pacinian corpuscle, sensory nerve, adipose tissue, vein, artery
Q1. forearm
R1. lumbar
S1. front of elbow
T1. chest
U1. integumentary, skeletal, muscular, articular, nervous, circulatory, digestive, respiratory, urinary, reproductive, endocrine
V1. cheek
W1. wrist
X1. inferior portion of ventral body cavity below diaphragm encircled by abdominal wall, bones, and muscles of pelvis
Y1. back of hand
Z1. covers surfaces because cells are in contact, lines hollow organs, cavities and ducts, forms glands when cells sink under the surface
A2. thymus gland, heart, pericardial cavity, left lung, horacic aorta, left pleural cavity, scapula
B2. navel
C2. neck

___ 32. olecranal
___ 33. crural
___ 34. phalangeal
___ 35. dorsum
___ 36. facial
___ 37. Cellular level integument
___ 38. dorsal
___ 39. anterior
___ 40. abdominopelvic cavity organs
___ 41. acromial
___ 42. Systemic Anatomy
___ 43. melanocyte distinguish
___ 44. orbital
___ 45. occipital
___ 46. cervical
___ 47. Systemic Anatomy definition
___ 48. buccal
___ 49. pedal
___ 50. abdominopelvic cavity location
___ 51. mental
___ 52. mediastinum's organs
___ 53. otic
___ 54. plantar
___ 55. scapular
___ 56. inguinal
___ 57. Connective
___ 58. digital
___ 59. posterior
___ 60. merkel cell distinguish
___ 61. trunk
___ 62. palmar
___ 63. thoracic cavity organs left side, anterior to posterior

D2. armpit
E2. calf
F2. heel
G2. groin
H2. thigh
I2. shoulder lade
J2. melanin granule
K2. leg
L2. ankle
M2. hand
N2. towards the front
O2. between hips
P2. eye
Q2. encircled by ribs, sternum, vertebral column, muscle divided into two pleural cavities by mediastinum
R2. thymus gland, heart, pericardial cavity, thoracic aorta, left pleural cavity, scapula, sternum, muscle, pericardium, right pleura, esophagus, sixth thoracic veertebra, rib
S2. fingers or toes
T2. shoulder
U2. tissues that bind together; cells rarely touch due to extracellular matrix; matrix (fibers & ground substance secreted by cells), consistency varies: liquid, gel, &solid; Doesn't occur on free surface, good nerve & blood supply except cartilage & tendons
V2. palm
W2. mouth
X2. nose
Y2. back
Z2. chin
A3. back of elbow
B3. anterior surface of knee
C3. intermediate filament, keratin
D3. towards the back
E3. keratinocyte, melanocyte, langerhans cell, merkel cell, sensory neuron
F3. standing upright, facing the observer, eyes facing forward, feet flat on floor, arms at sides, palms turned forward
G3. base of skull
H3. hollow behind knee
I3. spinal column
J3. skull
K3. face
L3. liver, diaphragm, stomach, gallbladder, large intestine, abdominal cavity, pelvic cavity, small intestine, urinary bladder

___ 64. Anatomical
___ 65. calcaneal
___ 66. femoral
___ 67. manual
___ 68. tissue level integument

M3. breastbone
N3. fingers
O3. sole
P3. sternum, muscle, pericardium, right lung, right pleura, esophagus, sixth thoracic vertebra, right pleural cavity, rib

Anatomy Test

Enter the letter for the matching Term

1. ☐ occipital
2. ☐ axillary
3. ☐ pedal
4. ☐ cervical
5. ☐ thoracic cavity organs left side, anterior to posterior
6. ☐ thoracic cavity location
7. ☐ otic
8. ☐ Tissues
9. ☐ calcaneal
10. ☐ orbital
11. ☐ posterior
12. ☐ acromial
13. ☐ brachial
14. ☐ sacral
15. ☐ Connective
16. ☐ Cellular level integument
17. ☐ mediastinum's organs
18. ☐ patellar
19. ☐ coxal
20. ☐ tissue level integument

A. encircled by ribs, sternum, vertebral column, muscle divided into two pleural cavities by mediastinum

B. epithelial, connective, muscle, nervous

C. ear

D. stratum corneum, dead keratinocytes, stratum lucidum, stratum granulosum, lamellar granules, stratum spinosum, langerhans cell, melanocytes, stratum basale, merkel cell, tactile disc, sensory neuron, dermis, blood vessel

E. neck

F. tissues that bind together; cells rarely touch due to extracellular matrix; matrix (fibers & ground substance secreted by cells), consistency varies: liquid, gel, &solid; Doesn't occur on free surface, good nerve & blood supply except cartilage & tendons

G. shoulder

H. thymus gland, heart, pericardial cavity, thoracic aorta, left pleural cavity, scapula, sternum, muscle, pericardium, right pleura, esophagus, sixth thoracic veertebra, rib

I. heel

J. armpit

K. towards the back

L. between hips

M. foot

N. arm

O. base of skull

P. anterior surface of knee

Q. eye

R. thymus gland, heart, pericardial cavity, left lung, horaic aorta, left pleural cavity, scapula

S. keratinocyte, melanocyte, langerhans cell, merkel cell, sensory neuron

T. hip

Give the Term that corresponds to the displayed Definition.

21. buccal

22. scapular

Give the Definition that corresponds to the displayed Term.

23. lying face up

24. thigh

25. standing upright, facing the observer, eyes facing forward, feet flat on floor, arms at sides, palms turned forward

26. towards the front

27. calf

28. back of elbow

29. dermal papilla, capillary loop, sweat pore, sebaceous gland, meissner copuscle, arrector pili muscle, hair follicle, hair root, eccrine sweat gland, pacinian corpuscle, sensory nerve, adipose tissue, vein, artery

30. toes

Anatomy Quiz

Circle the letter of the Term that corresponds to the displayed Definition.

1. otic

    A. spinal column

    B. anterior surface of knee

    C. ear

    D. stratum corneum, dead keratinocytes, stratum lucidum, stratum granulosum, lamellar granules, stratum spinosum, langerhans cell, melanocytes, stratum basale, merkel cell, tactile disc, sensory neuron, dermis, blood vessel

2. antecubital

    A. front of elbow

    B. toes

    C. forearm

    D. calf

3. popliteal

    A. lying face down

    B. hollow behind knee

    C. calf

    D. chest

4. crural

    A. top of foot

    B. hip

    C. leg

    D. toes

5. thoracic cavity organs right side, anterior to posterior

    A. dermal papilla, capillary loop, sweat pore, sebaceous gland, meissner copuscle, arrector pili muscle, hair follicle, hair root, eccrine sweat gland, pacinian corpuscle, sensory nerve, adipose tissue, vein, artery

    B. leg

    C. base of skull

    D. sternum, muscle, pericardium, right lung, right pleura, esophagus, sixth thoracic vertebra, right pleural cavity, rib

6. mediastinum's organs

    A. back of elbow

    B. thymus gland, heart, pericardial cavity, thoracic aorta, left pleural cavity, scapula, sternum, muscle, pericardium, right pleura, esophagus, sixth thoracic veertebra, rib

    C. dermal papilla, capillary loop, sweat pore, sebaceous gland, meissner copuscle, arrector pili muscle, hair follicle, hair root, eccrine sweat gland, pacinian corpuscle, sensory nerve, adipose tissue, vein, artery

    D. toes

7. plantar
    A. eye
    B. hollow behind knee
    C. ankle
    D. sole

8. dorsum
    A. palm
    B. back of hand
    C. neck
    D. lying face down

9. dorsal
    A. between hips
    B. chin
    C. back
    D. back of elbow

10. posterior
    A. epithelial, connective, muscle, nervous
    B. hollow behind knee
    C. spinal column
    D. towards the back

Circle the letter of the Definition that corresponds to the displayed Term.

11. lying face up
    A. Supine
    B. digital
    C. Systemic Anatomy definition
    D. merkel cell distinguish

12. keratinocyte, melanocyte, langerhans cell, merkel cell, sensory neuron
    A. Cellular level integument
    B. loin
    C. Tissues
    D. tarsal

13. tissues that bind together; cells rarely touch due to extracellular matrix; matrix (fibers & ground substance secreted by cells), consistency varies: liquid, gel, &solid; Doesn't occur on free surface, good nerve & blood supply except cartilage & tendons
    A. otic
    B. Connective

C. scapular
D. pedal

14. chest
    A. tarsal
    B. digital
    C. frontal
    D. thoracic

15. organization of body into organ systems
    A. antecubital
    B. nasal
    C. thoracic cavity location
    D. Systemic Anatomy definition

16. spinal column
    A. vertebral
    B. Connective
    C. crural
    D. thoracic

17. neck
    A. integumentary system
    B. femoral
    C. cervical
    D. tarsal

18. hip
    A. keratinocyte distinguish
    B. coxal
    C. scapular
    D. loin

19. arm
    A. axillary
    B. frontal
    C. antebrachial
    D. brachial

20. intermediate filament, keratin
    A. facial
    B. Systemic Anatomy

C. Epithelial
D. keratinocyte distinguish

EXTRA CREDIT: Give the Definition that corresponds to the displayed Term.

21. epithelial, connective, muscle, nervous

Printed in Great Britain
by Amazon